Troy's Tics

Explaining Tourette's Syndrome to Kids

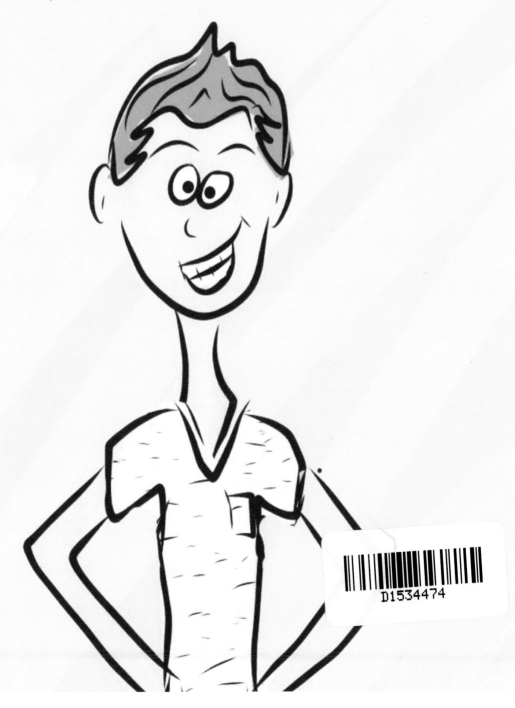

Written and Illustrated by:

Amy Marie Wells

Dedicated to my AMAZING son

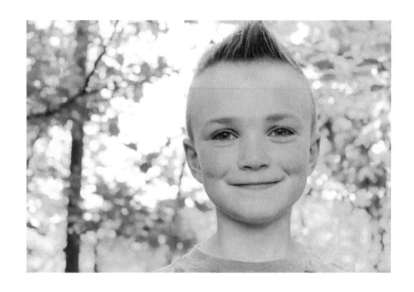

Troy Hunter Rohn

Troy's Tics

Explaining Tourette's Syndrome to Kids

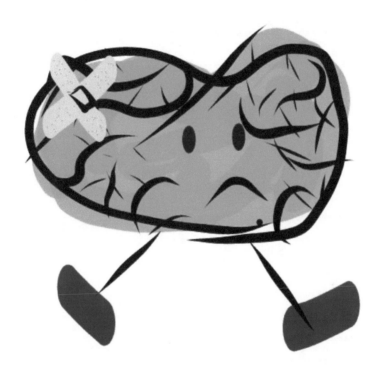

Written and Illustrated by Amy Marie Wells

This story is about an awesome boy. He is a normal kid just like you.

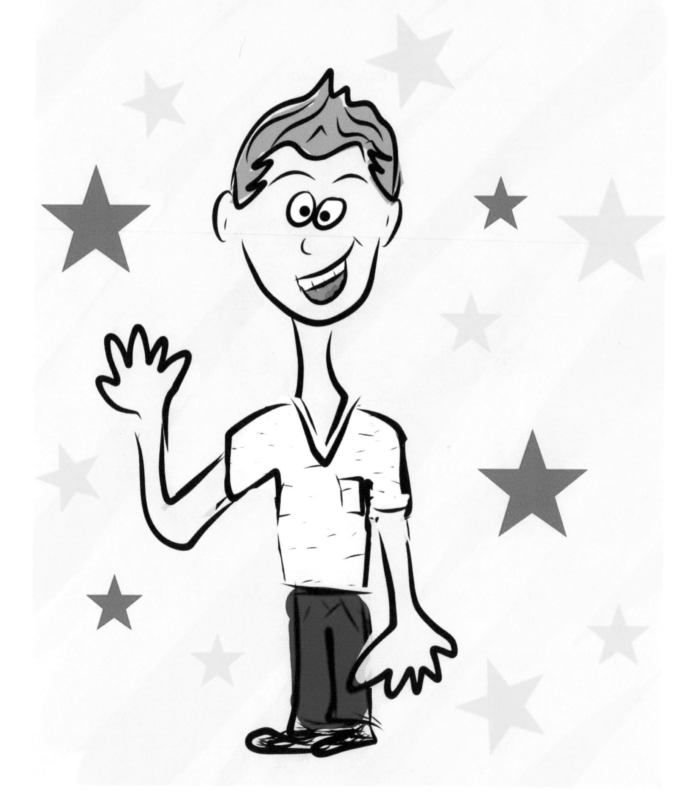

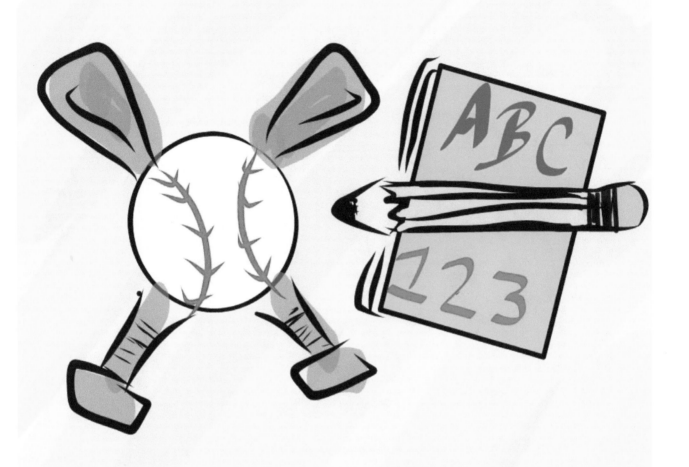

There is so many amazing things this awesome boy can do.

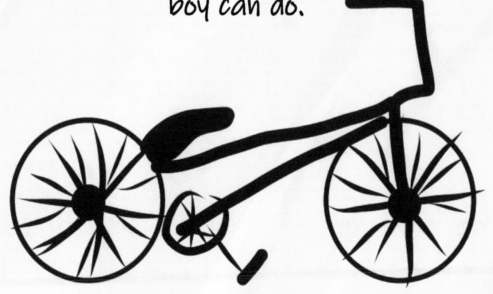

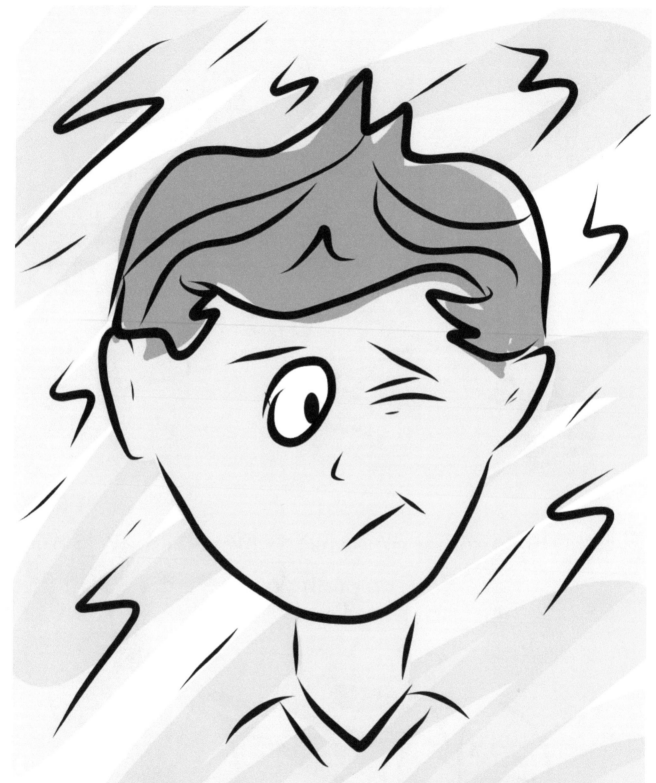

This boy's name is Troy, and sometimes his handsome face might make a twitch.

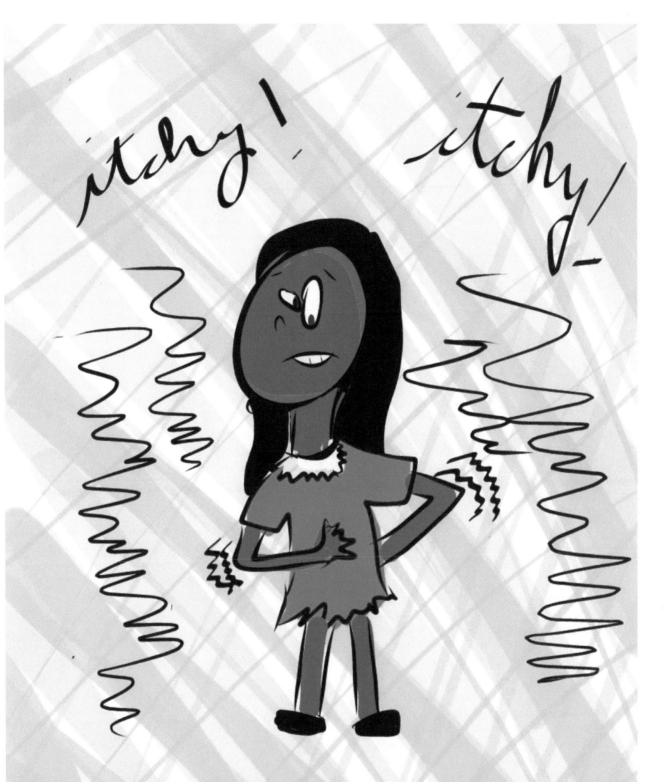

It is something he feels like he has to do, just like you have to scratch an itch.

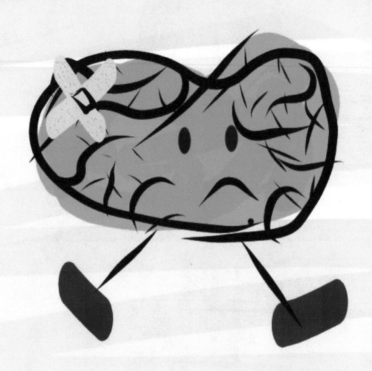

It all starts in his brain, and it's something he can not control.

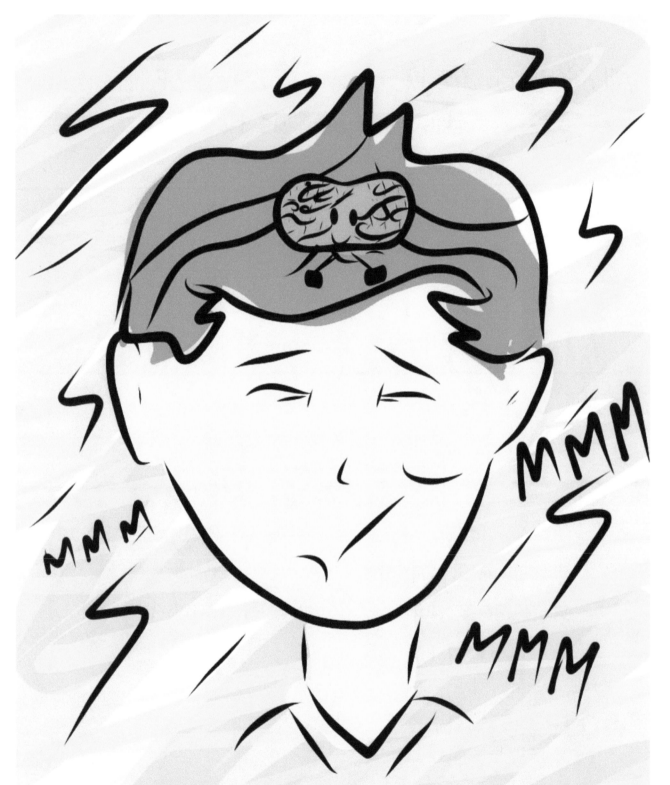

Humming, blinking, making a noise, or his eyes will have to roll.

All of these are just naming a few of the many things known as tics.

Motor Tics.

- Eye blinking.
- Rolling the eyes.
- Grimacing.
- Shaking head.
- Twitching shoulders.
- Twitching body.
- Movement of hands.

Vocal Tics.

- Coughing.
- Throat Clearing.
- Sniffing.
- Whistling.
- Grunting.
- Humming.
- Repeating words.

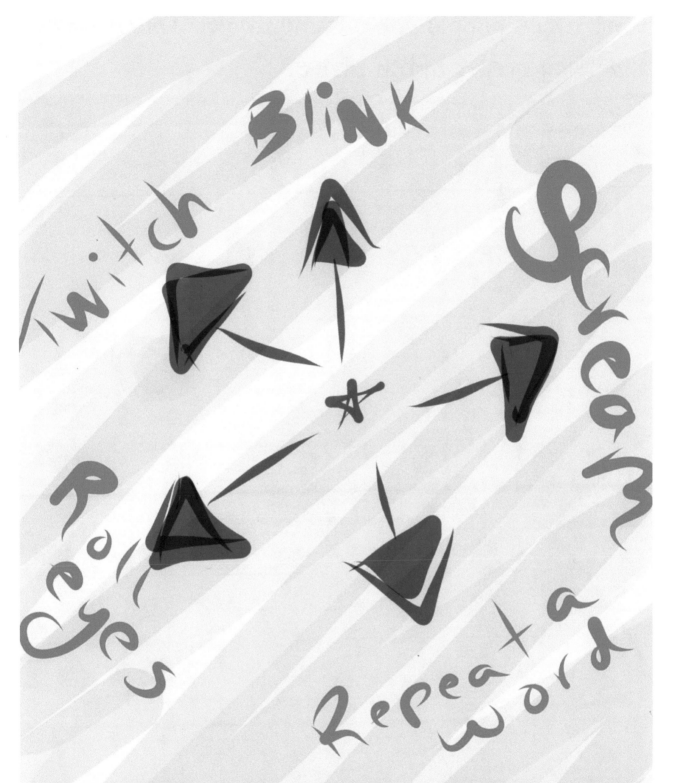

When someone has Tourette's Syndrome, they never know what tics they will get.

Sometimes people don't know about Tourette's, and they might often stare.

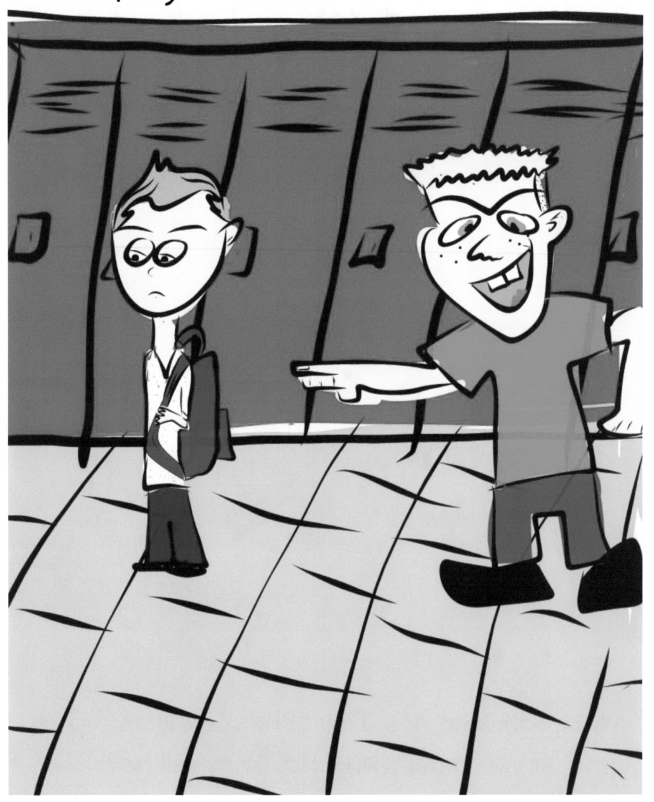

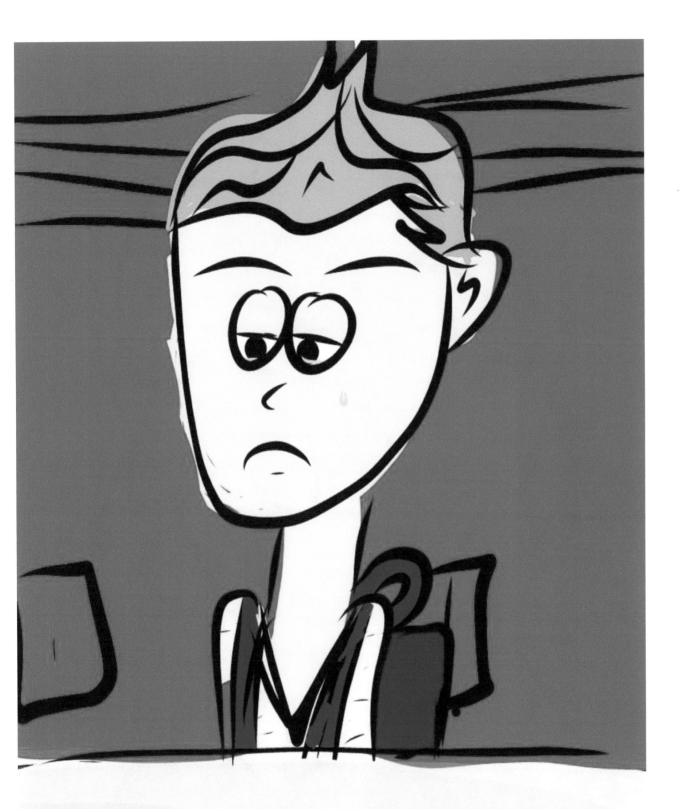

This might hurt Troy's feelings and make him sad, and that just is not fair.

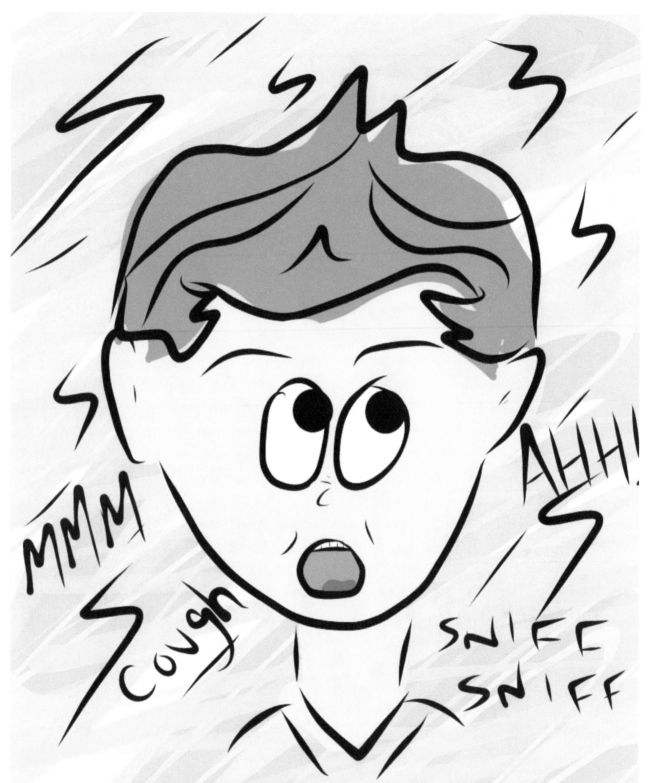

Troy's tics are always changing. He never knows what they will be.

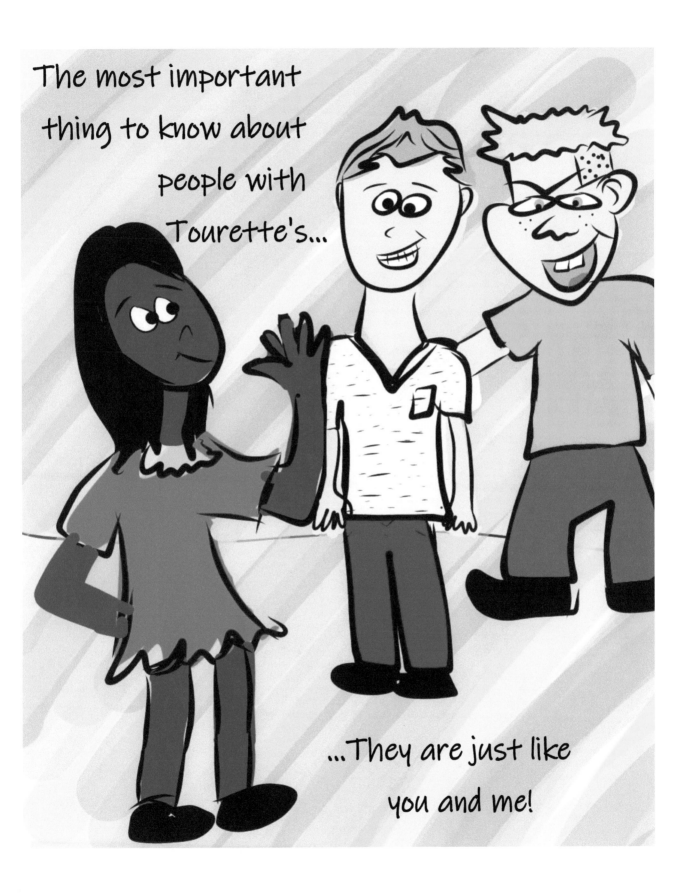

About Tourette's Syndrome

Tourette's Syndrome is something you are born with. Your brain is telling your body to do different things that you can't control. Almost anything can be a tic, and they're changing all the time! They can get worse when the person with Tourette's is anxious, excited, stressed, or nervous. They can calm down when the person is busy, and using their brain to do something else! Sometimes a person's tics will decrease once they're an adult, but some people have them their whole life.

How can I help someone with Tourette's?

People with Tourette's are just like you. The only thing they need is acceptance. They may need to make a face, sound, or whatever else their brain is telling them to do, but the best thing you can do is just ignore the tics, and treat them like anyone else!

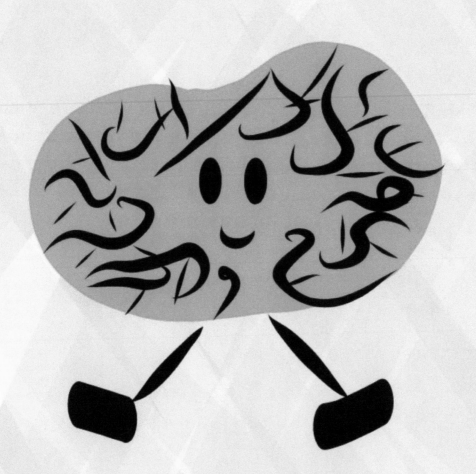

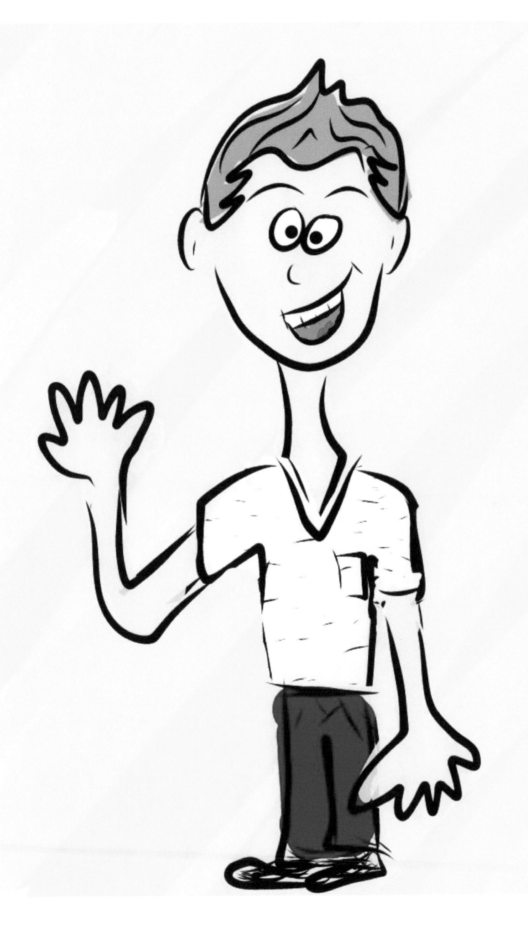

CPSIA information can be obtained
at www.ICGtesting.com
Printed in the USA
LVHW072336100919
630670LV00006B/24/P